Massage is a healing art that transcends the need for words. It takes you into a different world where time itself seems to stand still. It can make you feel a different person, in tune with nature and your own true self.

Here are some of the main benefits to be derived from a good massage:

Backache: We retain a lot of our past experiences in the form of backache. By rhythmically massaging the back muscles, particularly either side of the spine, toxins and deep-seated tensions from the past can be released and relieved. Simply resting in the 'Now' enables your partner to release the pain accumulated from the past.

Circulation: Is greatly improved and energy channelled to give a feeling of deep release and relaxation which heightens awareness and body power.

Constipation: This can be cured with regular, remedial massage and my *Wash Off Weight Formula Diet*. In a nutshell, this régime includes drinking a glass of hot water first thing in the morning and last thing at night. Eat regular meals of porridge with ripe bananas for breakfast; fresh fish, new potatoes with their skins and green salads for lunch, and wholemeal cake and herbal teas at tea time. For supper, have pasta, rice or cereal with vegetables; salad dressings should be made with pure olive oil and fresh herbs. Instead of dessert, fresh tropical fruits should be eaten first, before the meal.

Flatulence: The shaking and hacking movements in massage increase the vibrations that soothe the nerves of the alimentary tract which in turn relieves flatulence.

Fluid Retention: The lymphatic system is stimulated and is encouraged to disperse excess fluids.

Heart: The blood supply is increased threefold

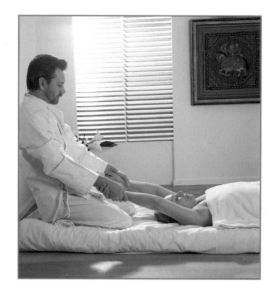

by the action of massage on the muscles and the consequent increase in the flow of nutrition to the muscle fibres and bones.

Indigestion: It is not a good idea to apply massage to your partner if they have eaten within the last two hours. However, massage is an excellent preventative of this complaint as it helps teach you to pace yourself and avoid rushing your food which would otherwise cause this problem.

Muscles: Are kept in tone and functional power increased, giving you greater elasticity and flexibility.

Nerves: The slow, rhythmical manipulation can produce sleep, by soothing the nerve endings.

Posture: Massage highlights and alerts you to your weak areas. You will soon realize that the areas causing you the most discomfort are the ones that have been neglected and misused

through poor posture. Taking time out to enjoy a massage gives you the ideal opportunity to reflect on how you are using and abusing your body.

Lack of Energy: Massage is a great restorative, a natural tonic for your glands and inner organs, and is especially beneficial for the production and distribution of the vital lymph flow.

Stress/Tension: It is so easy to become obsessed with the stress and strain of everyday life and regular treatment can help to channel these feelings, releasing tension from tight, tense muscles and stiff joints. It is possible to feel the benefits for up to a week afterwards. There is nothing finer than a little pampering and the loving attention derived from a treatment.

Headaches: You may sometimes find that you have a headache at the end of a treatment. This is because the stress rises. Avoid this by pulling the hair during a massage when I find that tensions are released which would otherwise cause the headache.

Skin: The tone and texture definitely improves. This is because the dead cells are exfoliated from the surface allowing the skin to more easily absorb the natural oils being massaged, making the skin more pliable and giving it a healthy glow.

Weight Problems: Cellulite is the bane of most women's lives. Regular massage with essential oils, accompanied by my *Wash Off Weight Formula,* will work wonders. Body weight is brought into balance because the body energies are harmonized and waste products eliminated through the gentle manipulation of the whole body during a massage treatment.

Emotions: Deep seated emotions such as anger, fear, frustration etc., can be released through remedial massage. It is important to allow your partner to cry should they feel the need.

PREPARING AROMATHERAPY OILS FOR MASSAGE

Aromatherapy massage has become increasingly popular over the last few years and there are courses running in most night schools. One of the reasons for its rise in popularity is that it has the added bonus of being a truly holistic treatment. It encompasses the whole individual, mind, body, emotion and spirit, treating the human organism in its entirety.

Before commencing treatment, a complete assessment of lifestyle, including eating habits and personal relationships, should to be taken into account. It is necessary to make a thorough study of the numerous therapeutic qualities of essential oils, for it is these oils, when blended with carrier/base oils, which will make up the 'treatment' to be tailored to your partner's individual needs.

Essential oils are derived from natural sources such as seed, flowers, fruit, peel, leaves, grass, roots, wood, bark and resins.

The primary purpose of carrier oils is as a means of lubrication for use in general massage or as a means of diluting essential oils. The reason for the dilution is that essential oils are far too concentrated in their original form and could cause irritation if applied directly to the skin.

Almost any pure vegetable oil such as soya, sunflower, or safflower can be used. These can be obtained from most supermarkets or health food stores. Sesame seed oil is probably one of the the most suitable as it can be easily washed out of sheets and towels. Here is an outline of the most popular carrier oils:

Rich and nourishing:
Peach and apricot kernel, avocado: these are excellent for dry and ageing skin.

Healing: Olive oil for extra dry skin, e.g. psoriasis. Wheatgerm oil (rich in vitamin E) is an anti-scarring agent and needs to be blended with lighter oils, such as almond, on a 25 to 75 per cent ratio.

Light: Grapeseed, grapefruit or orange. These are excellent light oils which can be used on most skins.

AVOID: Mineral or baby oils. They are unsuitable for this purpose and clog up the surface of the skin.

Blending Essential and Carrier Oils

In general terms, you would expect to dilute your chosen essential oil(s) in a 3% solution with your carrier oil. This amounts to 3 drops of essential oil(s) to 5ml of carrier oil. Either use a glass dispensing jug purchased from a chemist or a 5ml medicine-dispensing spoon. For calculating quantities suitable for your partner, see section on estimating quantities below.

Important Note: It must be remembered that a blend of essential oils and its carrier oil is primarily a 'treatment'. The method of delivery, i.e. massage, is strictly the secondary consideration. Dosage can be quite crucial when dealing with a number of medical conditions and when your partner is vulnerable, sensitive, or in a distressed state.

Buying, Preparing & Storing Oils

1. Buy the best possible organic oils from a reputable company for the very best results. Cheap oils are a false economy. Look for 'Pure Essential Oil' on the label, not 'Essence'.
2. Check they are environmentally friendly, non-animal tested and produced solely from plants and their by-products.
3. Certificates of purity are available on request. A reputable company will guarantee pure and economical products, e.g. Neal's Yard of Covent Garden, London.
4. Don't be taken in by fancy packaging.
5. If you find all your oils are the same colour then they are not pure oils. They should also vary in price from one to another.
6. Smell essential oils by testing on a handkerchief. If the smell evaporates quickly it is not a pure essential oil. Cultivate your natural intuition and senses to help you buy the best. Train your sense of smell and touch.
7. Don't be afraid to question your retailer and to ask for written information on the products.
8. Test oils for texture. If it is too viscous, leaving an oily residue on the skin, then it has had a vegetable oil added.

Storing:

1. Keep tightly sealed to prevent evaporation and deterioration through oxidation.
2. Store in a cool dark place out of direct sunlight and at an even temperature.
3. Plastic bottles will only keep oils in good conditions for up to eight weeks. Use dark brown or blue glass bottles.
4. Keep out of the reach of children and animals. Most of these oils are highly toxic if ingested.
5. Most oils, except sandalwood, cedarwood, vetiver, patchouli and rose otto can be stored in a fridge.
6. Most essential oils have a shelf life of about two years if kept in their pure state, i.e. unblended. They go cloudy as they become stale. Citrus oils have a six month shelf life, so buy in smaller quantities. Bergamot lasts well, neroli for up to one year, whereas patchouli and myrrh actually improve with age.

What You Need:

1. A small glass measuring/dispensing jug (from chemists) or 5ml medicine-dispensing spoon for accurately measuring carrier oils.
2. A glass eye-dropper to dispense essential oils.
3. A glass container or glazed ceramic bowl for mixing (optional).
4. Wooden or ceramic implement (miniature spatula, spoon etc.) for stirring/blending (optional).
5. Dark-tinted glass bottles for storage.
6. Self-adhesive labels and permanent (oil-proof) marker/pen for labelling formulas and partner identification.

Estimating Quantities:

A standard 5ml medicine-dispensing spoon (freely available) holds exactly 100 drops of oil. Most essential oils are used in a 3% solution. This means three drops of essential oil should be added to a 5ml spoonful of chosen carrier oil(s). Obviously one spoonful is not enough for an average adult massage, so I recommend the following proportions:

a) Baby (up to 6 months old, average size)
= 1 drop of essential oil to 5ml of a light carrier oil.
b) Child (up to 8 years old, average size)
= 2 drops of essential oil to 10ml.
c) Child (from 8-14 years old, average size)
= 3 drops of essential oil to 10ml.
d) Adult (small)
= 6 drops of essential oil to 10ml.
e) Adult (medium)
= 7-8 drops of essential oil to 15ml.
f) Adult (large)
= 9-10 drops of essential oil to 20ml.

Preparing a Massage Oil:

Step 1. Check contra-indications guidelines (see page 19)

Step 2. Choose appropriate:
a) Carrier oil(s)
b) Essential oil formula (see Page 13)
c) Quantities (see above)

Step 3. Wash and rinse your hands in clean running water, scrub nails thoroughly and dry on a clean towel.

Step 4. Working on a clean, stain-resistant surface, measure required quantity of carrier oil(s) into the dispensing jar or 5ml medicine spoon. Using either the built-in dropper, or your own eye-dropper, add prescribed number of drops of essential oil(s). Check smell and test texture of oils before using in case they have combined with oxygen and turned rancid, hardened, or lost freshness. Mix with wooden spatula.

Step 5. Decant into a clean dark-tinted bottle and shake gently to blend.

Step 6. Pour into a warmed, glazed ceramic bowl, clam shell or similar and warm your hands in preparation.

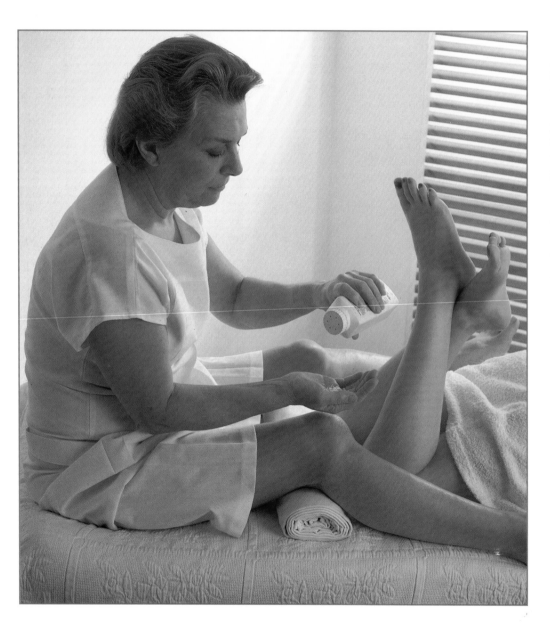

A part from base or carrier oils, which we have already discussed, there are other preparations which are useful aids to massage when for one reason or another an alternative is indicated.

Preparing a Massage Lotion for Face or Body
For those people who prefer the feel of a lotion rather than a vegetable-based oil, or are allergic or sensitive to certain products, a hypo-allergenic, non-perfumed, lanolin-free lotion can be used as a base.

Talcum Powders
Any talcum powder can be used (usually on the feet or hands) for reflexology-type treatments. Plain baby powder is a great favourite of mine, but there are lots of different herbal talcum powders available such as rosemary, sage, lavender, etc. Special fungicidal powders for problem feet, i.e. athlete's foot, can be used instead of standard talcum powders. Either sprinkle the powder onto your hands, rub them together, and smooth onto the skin or, alternatively, sprinkle directly onto the feet or hands.

Body Scrubs
These are excellent preliminaries or alternatives to the more traditional aromatherapy massage. They can be mixed with or without essential oils. My home recipes (see page 22) work wonders on the skin and have the added bonus of improving the whole circulation. They remove all the dead cells leaving the skin wonderfully smooth and silky.

On that fateful day when you stare into the mirror at a lined and haggard stranger, wondering whether you could possibly justify the cost of a face lift, you may seriously have to consider some form of 'damage limitation'.

First the good news. It doesn't take plastic surgery to achieve youthful features, just a few basic techniques that will make you the envy of your friends.

Start with a smile – it's the finest face-lift and will not only raise your spirits but the hearts of those around you. Acknowledge those lines of experience that have given your face its special character, you've earned them! Confidence and feeling good about yourself is the first rule of beauty care. It is not narcissistic but perfectly natural to wish to look your best at all times.

Contrary to what the media would have us believe, it is interesting to find just how liberating it is to discover your own natural self. Others feel much more at ease with a person who has no need to hide behind a painted mask. My mother seems to grow younger every day. She does not buy expensive cosmetics or formulas, she just lives at peace with herself. She has never ever sunbathed, so her skin has maintained its ability to produce natural oils. Skin that is well cared for may well be lined but it can still retain that glow of vitality that makes a woman attractive well into old age.

Premature wrinkling is caused by inner conflict. All the tension and worry you have experienced in your life may well start to show in your face. Your inner self is unfolding before your very eyes. Ultimately, only by resolving physical, emotional and mental imbalances will you notice improvement. Once you have learned to honestly confront the realities of your life, even the deepest worry lines will fade.

You will look and feel so much healthier if you undertake regular, natural treatments. Body massage and daily routines of slow rhythmical exercises such as yoga, regular deep relaxation, prayer or meditation will feed your inner self. I have found these are the most important preventative measures with which to combat the malaises of everyday life.

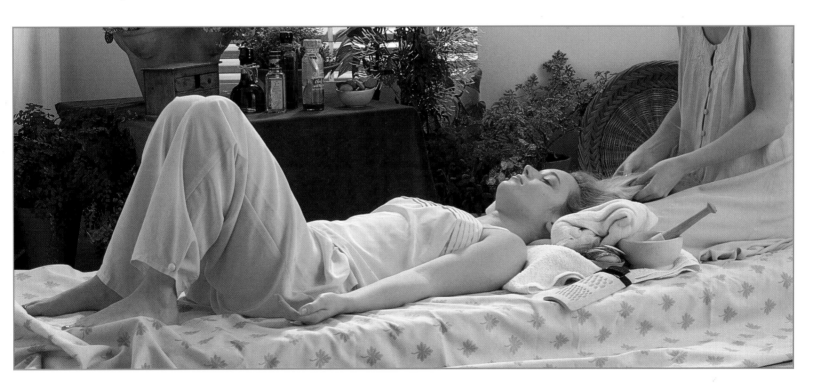

Step 1 Hair Combing (*Previous page*). Have your partner relax on their back, knees bent or resting on a pillow, feet in line with hips, arms lying freely by their sides (or resting palms on solar plexus), palms uppermost, fingers curling naturally. Place the neck on a rolled towel covered with an oblong piece of cheesecloth.

Gently draw all the hair away from the head, running your fingers through it for 2-3 minutes.

Aromatherapy Note (optional): Put 4 neat drops of essential oil in a line along the centre of the cheesecloth strip. Let your partner choose between lavender, rose, basil, melissa, lemongrass or peppermint (all excellent for headache/stress relief) or camomile, jasmine, neroli, petitgrain or ylang ylang as a general relaxant/refresher.

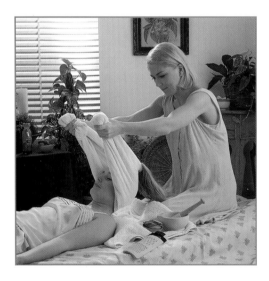

Step 2 *Above.* **Neck Stretch**
Take hold of the ends of the cheesecloth and lift your partner's head as far forward, chin towards the chest, as is comfortable. Hold for a second or two, then slowly and gently lower the head. Repeat several times, making sure the head is really relaxed and is cradled by the cloth. If you wish your partner to relax into this position it is imperative that they trust your skill and support.

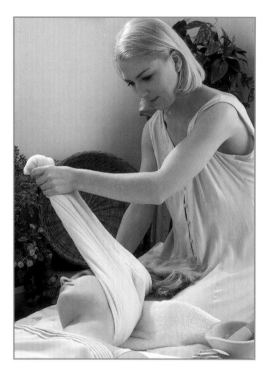

Step 3 *Above.* **Neck Extension**
With the head resting on the bed, pull up the left side of the cheesecloth over to the right, rolling the neck as far over to the right as is comfortable for your partner. Hold for a second or two then, lifting the right side of the cheesecloth, roll the head over to the left. Repeat slowly several times so that the head rolls freely from one side to the other.

Note: Step 2 & 3 can be repeated by cradling your partner's head in a pillow and then in your hands without a pillow underneath.

Caution: Keep the crown of the head centred on the base of the spine in all the movements.

Step 4 *Below.* **Hair Knot**
This simple technique can often relieve a tension-induced headache in a few minutes. If your partner has long hair, then weave it into the folds of the cloth in this technique. If your partner has short hair, then let the cloth do all the work. Explain, in advance, what you are going to do, and why. Ask for feedback so that you do not hurt them. It does, however, need to be firmly managed for full effect.

Cross the ends of the cloth over the brow, then fold the ends around the hair, slowly twisting and squeezing the knot tighter and tighter. Ask your partner to breathe out as you turn the knot and 'pull' the 'tension' out of the head. Hold for about 10-15 seconds. Slacken the hold and then repeat 2-3 times. Unravel the cloth from the hair and smooth out hair and cloth for the next step.

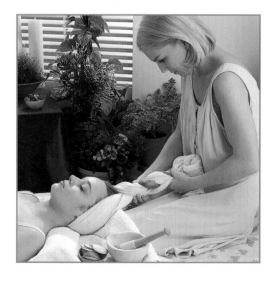

Step 5 *Below.* **Brow Smoothing**
Using either one end of the cheesecloth or a separate piece, press down on the brow and hold for approximately ten seconds. Release the pressure and repeat 2-3 times. Very gently stroke the cloth from eyebrows to hairline, repeating 3-4 times to soothe the lines of worry away.

Step 6 *Right.* **Face, Chest & Neck Smoothing**
Placing the cheesecloth strip down the right side of your partner's face (adjacent to the nose), smooth outwards to the outer edge of the face. Repeat 3-4 times on both sides. Then place the cloth across the chest and gently smooth upwards to a point under the chin. Repeat 3-4 times.

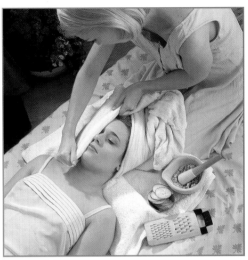

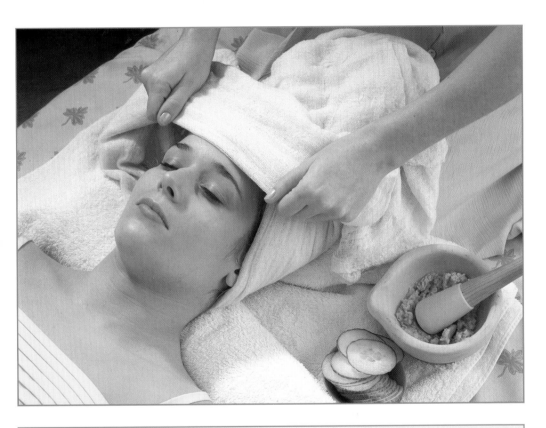

Step 7 *Below.* **Facial Scrub Treatment**
Blend together 2 tablespoons of Fuller's Earth with one tablespoon of fine children's play sand, or finely chopped nuts, and add enough rose or orange flower water to make a smooth paste. Gently rub the mixture into the face, avoiding the orbits of the eyes, lips and ears. Leave to set for 10 minutes. Cover with finely sliced cucumber. Leave for a further five minutes. Remove cucumber and wash off the scrub with warm water (scented with a few drops of flower water – optional) and a face flannel. Dry with a piece of cheesecloth by pressing gently onto the face.

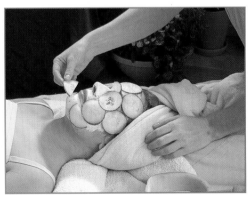

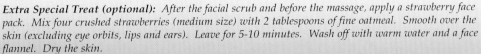

Extra Special Treat (optional): After the facial scrub and before the massage, apply a strawberry face pack. Mix four crushed strawberries (medium size) with 2 tablespoons of fine oatmeal. Smooth over the skin (excluding eye orbits, lips and ears). Leave for 5-10 minutes. Wash off with warm water and a face flannel. Dry the skin.
Massage: Using evening primrose oil or Vitamin E carrier oil, massage the face from chin to brow with small circular movements of your fingertips.
Finishing Touch: Dip your forefinger into flower water and dab on a point just between and above the eyebrows (third eye – tilak).

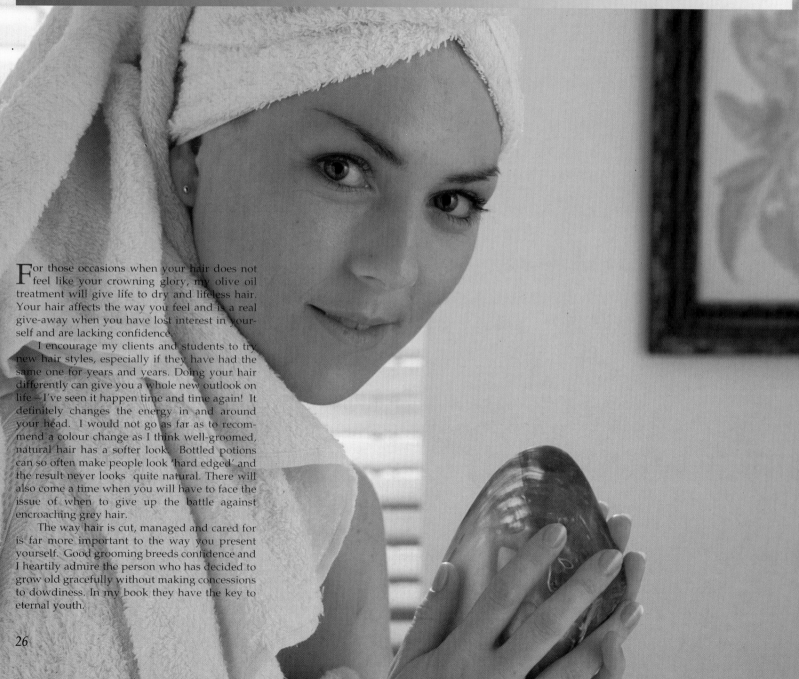

HAIR CARE
Natural Treatments to Enrich and Nourish

For those occasions when your hair does not feel like your crowning glory, my olive oil treatment will give life to dry and lifeless hair. Your hair affects the way you feel and is a real give-away when you have lost interest in yourself and are lacking confidence.

I encourage my clients and students to try new hair styles, especially if they have had the same one for years and years. Doing your hair differently can give you a whole new outlook on life ~ I've seen it happen time and time again! It definitely changes the energy in and around your head. I would not go as far as to recommend a colour change as I think well-groomed, natural hair has a softer look. Bottled potions can so often make people look 'hard edged' and the result never looks quite natural. There will also come a time when you will have to face the issue of when to give up the battle against encroaching grey hair.

The way hair is cut, managed and cared for is far more important to the way you present yourself. Good grooming breeds confidence and I heartily admire the person who has decided to grow old gracefully without making concessions to dowdiness. In my book they have the key to eternal youth.

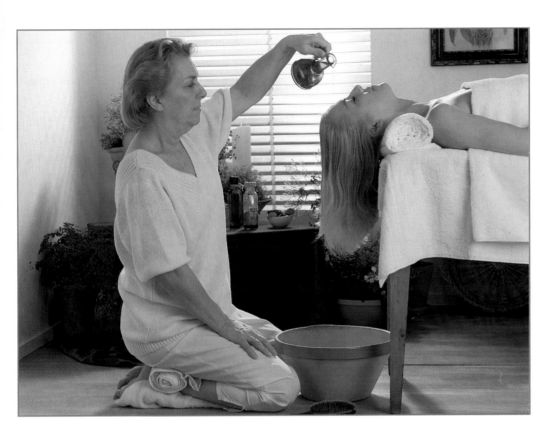

Step 2 *Below.* **Combing & Scalp Massage** Whether you partner's hair is long or short, run your fingers through the hair and scalp to work the oil in, massaging the oil thoroughly into the scalp and hair.

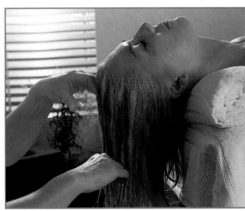

Step 3 *Below.* **Wringing (long hair)** If your partner has long hair, lightly squeeze off the surplus oil by wringing out the hair in your hands.

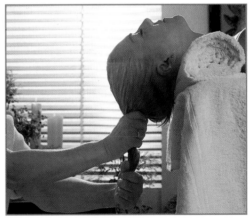

Step 4 *Not shown.* **Hot Towel Treatment**
Wrap a warm towel around the head. Let your partner rest for at least 30 minutes to enable the oils to penetrate the hair and scalp. Remove the towel and wash the hair in a mildly astringent shampoo of your choice. Rinse well, towel, and allow to dry without using a hairdryer.

Step 1 *Above.* **Applying the Olive Oil**
Firstly, warm approximately 250ml of pure, extra virgin, cold pressed olive oil. The very best quality is required to assure the tonic aspect of this technique. Do not heat quickly or to a very high degree lest you destroy some of the natural properties of this very special commodity. It is vital that you test the temperature of the mixture on the back of your partner's hand so that they approve and are prepared for the application.

Have your partner rest on a padded table, their head slightly tilted back, their neck resting on (and supported by) a rolled towel. Place a large bowl on the floor to catch the flow of oil.

Carefully, and very slowly, trickle then pour the warm oil onto a point a little above and between the eyebrows. This is traditionally recognized by some cultures as the site of the third eye and is the location of the vestigial pineal gland. The oil will flow over the brow, through the hair and onto the scalp. This is a blissful experience! The uniquely enjoyable aspect of the treatment is the sense of deep relaxation that is felt as the oil cascades over the head.

Note: *To help maintain healthy hair, try to avoid drying out the natural oils with hairdryers, sunbathing, chemical colourants and perming solutions. Brushing the hair and scalp regularly helps to stimulate the scalp and balance its natural functioning.*

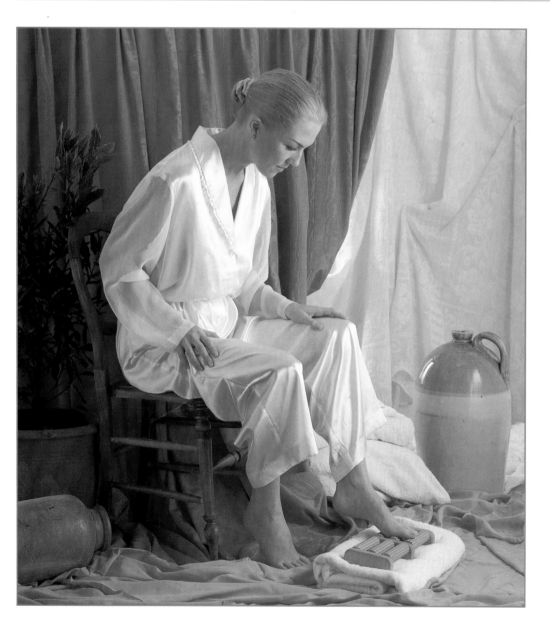

The following self-help treatments will prepare you for massage and maintain the health of your body. I use these wonderful wooden bath products which are available from many health shops. They can be used either under the shower or after a bath.

Rubbing the body with a rough bath towel is an excellent way of stimulating the circulation and removing any surplus dead skin, which can have an ageing effect if not removed. I feel quite strongly that it is important to wear loose-fitting clothes, made from natural fibres, in order to maintain a healthy skin. Tight-fitting, man-made fibres restrict the proper function of the skin and, I am quite convinced, cause a build-up of cellulite. Nylon underwear and stockings restrict the circulation and free movement of air around the body, marring freshness and natural cleanliness.

Step 1 *Left.* **Double Foot Roller**
Place both, or either of your feet on the ridged wooden rollers. Rub the feet forward and backwards as many times as you like with a pressure that suits your level of sensitivity.

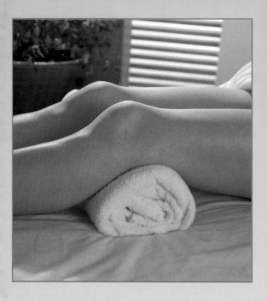

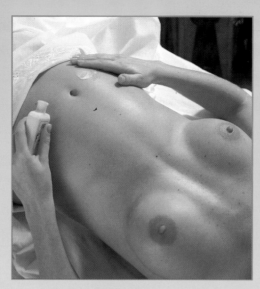

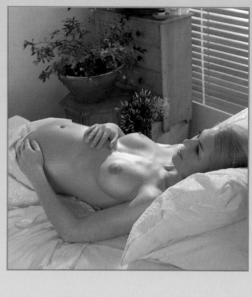

Step 1 Resting Position
Rest with a rolled bath towel under your knees and 3-4 pillows under your back, shoulders and head. The roll under the knees takes the pressure off the lumbar region.

Step 2 Oiling/Lotioning
Rub your selection of oils or lotions gently, in a clockwise direction around your abdomen and stomach until they have been absorbed by the skin. Then massage around each breast.

Step 3 Cradling & Comforting – 8 months
During the pregnancy, whilst the baby's head is uppermost, place your hands above and below its growing form. Visualize loving energies flowing between the poles of your palms and providing energetic nourishment.

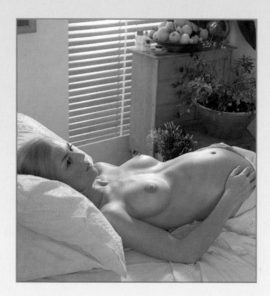

Step 4   Preparing for the Birth
When you have felt (or been informed) that the baby has turned and is head down, change the position of your hands and visualize a safe delivery.

I hope you have enjoyed learning and partaking in the language of touch. Keep practising in order that your loving relationships may be enhanced. Autograph all your work with excellence and continue to perfect your caring involvement with others.

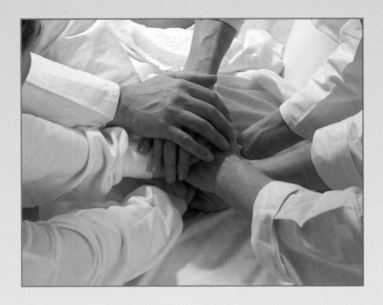